YOUR KNOWLEDGE HAS VALUE

AF136004

- We will publish your bachelor's and master's thesis, essays and papers

- Your own eBook and book - sold worldwide in all relevant shops

- Earn money with each sale

Upload your text at www.GRIN.com and publish for free

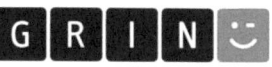

Health system and financial inequalities in the UK, Mexico and Ghana. An assessment of financing mechanisms for the promotion or reduction of health inequalities

Abdullah Adigun

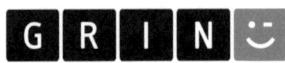

Bibliographic information published by the German National Library:

The German National Library lists this publication in the National Bibliography; detailed bibliographic data are available on the Internet at http://dnb.dnb.de.

ISBN: 9783346537911
This book is also available as an ebook.

© GRIN Publishing GmbH
Nymphenburger Straße 86
80636 München

All rights reserved

Print and binding: Books on Demand GmbH, Norderstedt, Germany
Printed on acid-free paper from responsible sources.

The present work has been carefully prepared. Nevertheless, authors and publishers do not incur liability for the correctness of information, notes, links and advice as well as any printing errors.

GRIN web shop: https://www.grin.com/document/1145708

Comparative and Critical Assessment of Financing Mechanisms for the Promotion or Reduction of Health Inequalities in the UK, Mexico and Ghana

Table of contents

Introduction

The World Health Report, 2000 recommends that the global health care system performances has to be assessed by the average health of the population as well as by how citizen's health status and the financial burden of health care is evenly distributed among the population. This dominant concern with equity is reflected in many modern directives on health, all in an attempt to present an equitable system without financial preference on a global scale. For individuals at the top of the socio-economic spectrum, the multiple mechanisms adopted by UK, Ghana and the Mexican health systems provide excellent care according to any standard. But for the citizens at the bottom of such social distributions, system delivers a little more than a vaccination. The objective of this report is to conduct a critical and comparative analysis of UK, Ghana and Mexican health system with special emphasis on financial inequalities discerned.

Financial Mechanisms in the UK

Minimizing health inequalities has been placed along with health gain as a pivotal point of governmental policy. Leading organizations including the Department of Health, Standards and Planning Framework with National Improvement Plan place an emphasis on need for healthcare organizations to set up joint partnership along with other agencies to reduce the rise of health inequalities (Ledger, 2017). UK government policy was narrowly aimed to address a wider range of determinant factors of health including; lifestyle, employment, housing, income, crime and environment in conjunction with actions across governments, community, voluntary and business sectors (Marmot, 2011). Public Service Announcement targets were dominated by government departments with relations to health inequalities, including ODPM;

improvement of social housing, transport; reduction in fatal accidents, provision of better employment while sinking poverty, etc (Turkentine, 2010).

With a GDP of 0.3 percent increase in total expenditure on health as since 1980 till 2019 (Elflein, 2020), the UK's approach to tackle health inequalities is divided in two:

i.   The Black Report and

ii. the Acheson Report.

As a result of the fact that these two are different with reference to their impacts they are vital in the establishment of a relationship between evidence and policy (Marmot, 2011). In 1997 in the UK, the Labour party published a report referred to as the Black Report (1980) regarding health inequalities for which 4 four determinants of were identified:

i.   Artefact

ii.   Natural selection

iii. Cultural

iv.   Structural

Despite the acclaimed comprehensiveness, it was observed that no mediation in healthcare was being conducted in order to reduce health inequalities (Ledger, 2017). The government in power rejected the report as a result of the high-costing proposals and opposition to the issue, as a result of which it had minimum impact on policy in over 10 years (Smith & Eltanani, 2015). Afterwards, the Acheson Report was designed to determine that scientific evidence supported socio-economic explanations of health inequality. (Marmot, 2011). As a result, the report collaborated environments including socio-economic factors and individual lifestyles. On the evaluation of its social determinants, it considered the following:

i.   Poverty

ii. Education

4

iii. Employment

iv. Housing

v. Transport

vi. Nutrition

vii. Ethnicity

viii. Gender

ix. Healthcare

It indicated 3 vital factors namely:

"All possible policies having impact on health should be analysed with regards to their impact on Health inequalities".

"High priority should be given to health of families with children".

Further steps are required to reduce income inequalities and improve standard of living in poor households" (Committee of Inquiry, 1988).

The Report was *welcomed* by the government, although it was not universal, several academics collaborated on the report which resulted into several criticisms (Bambra, et al., 2010);

i. **No Priorities**: Some recommendations carried equal-burden. According to Illsley (1999) "the recommendations were similar to a *shopping List.* "

ii. **No Mechanism:** The process in which policymakers renovate recommendations into actions were necessary. Thus, they were argued to be "politically naïve".

iii. **Evidence Policy Mismatch:** The absence of collaborating evidence between policy and application resulted into an undetermined report (Mackenbach, 2014).

iv. **Specificity of Recommendations**: family health of families including children and high-priority recommendations were unclear for policy-makers to implement

(Turkentine, 2010). Others were too distinguishing and no implementations were considered.

v. **Cost effectiveness:** The lack of evidence about cost-effectiveness resulted into concerns especially as a result of the absence of tackling of policies against inequalities. Therefore, it is important especially since the Black Report was rejected as a result of costly recommendations.

As a result, the adaptation of the newly adopted policies is associated with the recommendations following these criticisms.

The life-course initiative is the focus of the UK health inequality, in connection with early years of childhood which contains an explanatory approach (Bartley, 2016). The Sure Start initiative in UK was aimed for the improvement of the possibility of young children and families living in poor areas to experience a change in existing services. As a result, 500 programs were introduced in 2004 with an objective to reach $^1/_3$ of UK children in poverty. Due to this design, children in poverty somewhere else will not be considered for the benefits except the policy is converted from sure to unsure start area (Ledger, 2017).

In 2004, child poverty was the UK government's aim, with intent in reduction by ¼ since it has over past years been suffering from high rates of poverty (WHO, 2016). This was calculated according to households with incomes below 60% of the national median income. Implemented policies were targeted for individuals in disadvantaged communities; their contributions included increasing welfare benefits as well as incorporating benefits with impacts for low-paid workers and through the subsidization of child care (Turkentine, 2010). Research indicate that progress report regarding the matter was inconclusive, statistics however indicate that between 1996 and 2001, "there was a downfall of 1.3M in the amount of children below 60% of 1996-1997 median income" (Office for National Statistics, 2002). Besides the fact that it is impossible to attribute the identified changes to policies alone, children were raised from poverty-range in which nearest poverty line-resulted into a lack of residual group thereby making existing policies seem unreachable.

In 2003, Area-Based Initiatives in which UK was mainly focused on policies targeting close relation to geographical communities with an emphasis on poverty and its disadvantages were adopted. Such initiatives include:

Health Action Zone which was composed of companies through which 26 areas of poverty and deprivation in Health were acknowledged, with an astounding total coverage of about 13 million citizens (Ledger, 2017). The HAZ attempted to implement strategies organize with an objective to reduce health inequalities. It however, HAZ suffered from a continuous change in operation being founded in 1997. As a result of ulterior objectives, it is constantly employed by the government as a reform body in other sectors, which constituted a disadvantage for it.

As a result of its failure, the Redistribution-Welfare-to-Work provided a shift in concertation to poorer citizens across UK's social gradient (Black & Morris, 2013). Familiar forms of redistribution with an emphasis on taxation were designed, it used paid employment as an ideal escape for citizen poverty and connected benefit payments to employment in a scheme referred to as the "welfare-to-work". Other implemented policies combined minimum levels despite not being able to focus on inequality because they do not progressively redistribute (Mackenbach, 2014).

The implementation of UK's health policies has met with several criticisms, which has resulted into adoption and readoption of other policies. As a result of its fragmented society, it is difficult to find a policy which best suits its system, and this may enable the adoption of policies significant to individual environment at the expense of a national system.

Financial Mechanisms in Ghana

The national pattern of health finance globally depends on differing degrees of resources from national governments, private and social insurance, foreign bodies, non-governmental organizations, households and communities. Unlike in the case of the UK, Ghana has an unfortunate history of relying on a combination of rare government resources, donor-funded projects and high-levels of household contributions due to its under-developed nature. Due to an increase in budget deficits in the 1980s, a deterioration of both quantity and quality of public health services resulted in higher dependence on payments made by patients through the implementation of user fees which was supported both by the UNICEF and the World Bank (Gilson L, 2000). During the early 1990s, concerns were raised regarding the negative impacts of the fees on equity and access to healthcare (Castro-Leal, et al., 2014). As a result, Ghana gradually favoured the implementation of several financial mechanisms with an objective to reduce risks of disastrous payments (Adisah-Atta, 2017). In more recent times, there is significant attention towards innovative schemes designed to address health equity issues. Performance based contracts were introduced in an effort to improve efficiency and equity in the Ghanaian health sector in the supply department (Ekman, 2016), as well as demand incentives which were focused on poor people have been attracting an increased attention among policy-makers. It is worthy to note that the poorest Ghanaian population remain exempted from health care, this is including services established to be highly cost-effective which have begun to fail to reach the needy (Lagarde & Palmer, 2018). Along these lines, there is an increasing evidence regarding individuals with the least access who are the poorest and most vulnerable at the same (Preker & Carrin, 2011). As a result of these factors, a limited access as well as a low utilization of the important health services is contributory factors to the persistence of disease as well as a low life expectancy.

Ghana's GDP on health experienced an increase by 6.8% between 2017 and 2018, to 3.5 of its total economy (Adisah-Atta, 2017). It is important to note that the Ghanaian health care system unlike UK, is financed by both direct and indirect tax revenues (Bambra, et al., 2010). With reference to direct tax and personal-income tax, workers contribute a total of 5% of retirement income, an amount collected by the SSNIT; a social security organization (Castro-Leal, et al., 2014). These rates fall within 0% for incomes less than GH¢180 to a figure of 28% for incomes exceeding GH¢720 (Adisah-Atta, 2017). Personal tax is a contributor of about 5.2% health expenditure of the Ghanaian health system.

The heavy reliance of the Ghanaian system on tax enables corporate tax to feature as a funding source of the country's health system. The important elements of the debate regarding corporate tax is about whether an increase will lead to lower wages, low retail earnings, or higher prices. There is a general assumption an equal share of burden for customers and shareholders, while others argue for a 10% burden on customers and 90% on shareholders (Lagarde, et al., 2014). Besides these speculations, corporate tax contributes 7.1% to total health expenditure of Ghana. At the same time, Value Added Tax (VAT) is used to finance the health sector. Due to this, the current total rate of collected VAT is 15% (Adisah-Atta, 2017). This includes VAT component of 10% with additional sector components of 2.5% each.

Unlike the UK, Ghanaian fuel levy is another mechanism through which the country funds its health sector. In 2005, the levy was second to VAT in contribution to national total tax revenue, at 8.5% (Castro-Leal, et al., 2014). Ghana's fuel composition includes petrol, kerosene and diesel. Kerosene is consumed more citizens without a constant access to in remote areas. This has resulted into a high cost of kerosene which consumes a significant part of family's income. Due to the fact that kerosene is frequently purchased, it was annualized (Gilson L, 2000) resulting into more difficulties for these families. Besides the indicated sources, import duty is also a contributor to the finance of the Ghanaian health sector. It is the third largest contributor of tax after VAT and income tax for the Ghanaian economy. It contributes a total of 8.0%

health expenditure in Ghana, and apart from the tax, Ghanaian health care is financed by

contributions from health insurance comprising of premiums and pay roll deductions to the

(NHIS) National Health Insurance Scheme and out-of-pocket payments (OOP) (Ekman, 2016).

The design of the mechanisms influencing inequalities in the Ghanaian health sector seem to

be concentrated further towards increasing the gap in inequalities. As indicated, majority of the

revenue generated for health care in Ghana is through tax, which has a more negative influence

on Ghanaians than not. The only advantage is that the quality of the provided healthcare service

at least is impressive, but this is only because it rips off of the meagre income that a majority

of its poor population are able to garner. The system is therefore disadvantageous towards the

reduction of health inequality instead only expands it further as it implies that while the rich

are barely bothered, the country's poor population are enforced to pay a significant part of their

income in an effort to obtain health care services.

Financial Mechanisms in Mexico

With significant differences to Ghana and the UK, the structure and financing mechanisms of

Mexican healthcare system is a critical impediment to the reduction of health inequity. This is

in the midst of ensuring citizens are guaranteed equal access to basic package of health-care

services with protection from financial destruction as a negative effect of ill-health (Barraza-

Lloréns, et al., 2013). Mexican government preserves multiple, parallel systems for different

population categories, which create incentives for the maintenance or increase of inequity

rather than channelling resources into pressing needs (Danese-Dlsanto, 2011). Although the

UK and Ghanaian systems are different from Mexico's, an analogy indicates that inequity in

consistent to health care is observed due to the separation of the policies implemented.

Mexico's 100 million citizens receive health care from a system composed of 3 principal subsystems:

(1) social security institutes which provide health insurance for formally employed people and their families, such a system is financed by employer and employees payroll taxes including legally mandated contributions

(2) government services managed by the Ministry of Health as well as limited services from NGOs for uninsured Mexican citizens

(3) a huge private sector almost financed out-of-pocket because of the coverage of the private insurance market (Williamson A, 2020).

Closer to the American system, Mexico's social security sector encompasses different institutions which provide range of benefits for the advantage of different parts of its labour market. As the largest of the institutions, the Mexican Social Security Institute (IMSS) has an organizational structure similar to a huge, vertically integrated; staff modelled health maintenance organization (HMO). The IMSS was created in response to political pressures of emerging worker class in association with rapid industrialization (Urquieta-Salomón & Villarreal, 2015). The organization's funding mechanism has a foundation in mutual societies arranged by employees (Leslie, 2019). Since foundation, employers, employees, and federal government has contributed to its scheme. Access to health care was a significant aspect of these requirements, though it was created within welfare purposes: which includes the provision of workers with social security benefits, this includes coverage against health risks; provision of financial security benefits for retirement; and protection against financial loss which are associated with disabilities or death (Gutierrez, 2020).

Though affiliation with it is mandatory for citizens employed within the formal economy, exceptional voluntary insurance schemes are incorporated to recognize the necessity of the provision of access to social insurance for some workers outside of the formal employee-employer relationship (Barraza-Lloréns, et al., 2013). Thus, with the increase in formal employment, there is a corresponding increase in social security coverage enabling it to eventually cover a majority of the population. However, political pressure from interest groups stopped the integration of some population groups into the single social security scheme; to cate for them, multiple parallel social security schemes were created for other formally employed citizens, including those employed by the federal government, state-owned oil companies (PEMEX), and military (Williamson A, 2020). Consequentially, these institutions have developed health care infrastructures, self-sufficiently providing services for members through separate finance and delivery mechanisms.

In Mexico, health care accounts for 5.3% of Mexico's GDP as well as an average per-capita health spending of $520 (Barraza-Lloréns, et al., 2013). The social security sector is responsible for 33% of its total health spending while the Ministry health service represents 13%. While the Ministry of Health has been responsible health system stewardship, especially policy making, regulation, and information gathering, only a fraction of the country's hospitals have been certified with a limitation to physician quality. Therefore, while the social security institution may have been an applicable scheme on paper, it provides a potential for effectiveness and efficiency while presenting an opportunity to cater for the health of all citizens. It is however worthy to note that since the creation of the health institution, there has been no major changes yet undertaken in the structure of Mexico's health care system (Urquieta-Salomón & Villarreal, 2015). Consequentially, the system remained fractured hovering between citizens access to social security coverage alias the upper echelons and the uninsured. Thus, a disadvantage of the system is its complexity, as well as the fact that it is not cost effective, making it essentially difficult to manage.

Reducing Health Inequalities in Ghana: Recommendations

If equity is the objective of the Ghanaian health system, then policy and evaluation standpoints have to be long-term. Despite the speed in change of the finance of the tax system, it is possible to repair the decay demonstrated and achieve greater equity in health status. Empirical evidence suggests that it is not feasible to continue to implement the same policy on the poorer citizens, whose means of livelihood is taking a heavy toll. This is why it is important for the country to adopt a national health care system, one that is not based primarily on a private taxation–funded scheme. Private and social insurance schemes funded by local taxes have to be integrated and strengthened as a means for the purchase of comprehensive insurance amenities for the generality of the populace. While this will further improve the quality of health care, it will take the burden off citizens from private tax to public tax revenue sources. The single health insurance scheme is anticipated to explicitly cover an elementary package of health care for Ghanaians, delivery can be organized in ways to include private sector while ensuring that public-sector capacity is applied for patients' benefit. It is easy to integrate arrangements in which patients can decide providers, with information on their rights and benefits under the scheme. This system can improve social capital as long as choice is endorsed.

Conclusion

The report conducted a critical and comparative analysis of how finance mechanisms promote or reduce health inequalities in the UK, Ghana and Mexico. The report focused on Mexico, the UK and Ghana, expressively demonstrating how they differed as well as the effectiveness and shortcomings of their health mechanisms. It thereafter proceeded to provide recommendations for the Ghanaian mechanism as a result of its heavy reliance on private-income tax of a developing economy and suggested a more central system locally funded.

References

Adisah-Atta, I., 2017. Financing Health Care in Ghana: Are Ghanaians Willing to Pay Higher Taxes for Better Health Care?. *Social Sciences,* 17(2), pp. 1-19.

Bambra, C., Gibson, M. & Sowden, A., 2010. Tackling the wider social determinants of health and health inequalities: evidence from systematic reviews. *Commun Health,* 65(2), pp. 284-291.

Barraza-Lloréns, M., Bertozzi, S., González-Pier, E. & Gutiérrez, J. P., 2013. Addressing Inequity In Health And Health Care In Mexico. *Mexico: Health Affairs,* 21(3), pp. 46-56.

Bartley, M., 2016. *Health Inequality: An Introduction to Theories, Concepts and Methods.* Cambridge: Cambridge Polity Press.

Black, D. & Morris, J. S. C., 2013. *Inequalities in Health - Report of A Research Working Group.* London: DHSS.

Castro-Leal, F., Dayton, J., Demery, L. & Mehtra, K., 2014. Public spending on health care in Africa: do the poor benefit ?. *Bulletin of the World Health Organization,* 78(1), p. 66-74..

Committee of Inquiry, i. t. F. D. o. t. P. H. F., 1988. *Public health in England: Report of the Committee of Inquiry into the Future Development of the Public Health Function.* London: The Stationery Office.

Danese-Dlsanto, L., 2011. Analysis of changes in the association of income and the utilization of curative health services in Mexico between 2000 and 2006.. *BMC Public Health,* pp. 113-134.

Ekman, B., 2016. Community-based health insurance in low income countries: a systematic review of the literature. *Health Policy and Planning,* 19(5), p. 249-70.

Elflein, J., 2020. Healthcare expenditure as a share of GDP in the United Kingdom (UK) 1980-2019. *Statista.*

Gilson L, M. A., 2000. Health sector reforms in sub-saharan Africa: lessons of the last 10 years. *Health Policy,* p. 215-43.

Gutierrez, J., 2020. Advances and challenges on the path toward the SDGs: subnational inequalities in Mexico, 1990-2017.. *BMJ Glob Health,* pp. 122-135.

Lagarde, M., Haines, A. & Palmer, N., 2014. The impact of conditional cash transfers on health outcomes and use of health services in low and middle income countries. *Cochrane Database of Systematic Reviews,* pp. 134-145.

Lagarde, M. & Palmer, N., 2018. The impact of health financing strategies on access to health services in low and middle income countries. *Cochrane Database Syst Rev. ,* 13(2), pp. 112-124.

Ledger, J., 2017. *Uk Policy Addressing Health Inequalities Health And Social Care.* London: Routledge.

Leslie, H., 2019. Assessing health system performance: effective coverage at the Mexican Institute of Social Security.. *Health Policy Plan,* pp. 16-25.

Mackenbach, J., 2014. Has the English strategy to address health inequalities failed?. *Soc Sci Med,* 71(2), pp. 1249-1253.

Marmot, M., 2011. *Strategic Review of health inequalities in England post,* London: London University College.

Office for National Statistics, 2002. *Census 2002*. London: Office for National Statistics.

Preker, A. & Carrin, G., 2011. *Health Financing for Poor People: Resource Mobilization and Risk Sharing.*, s.l.: World Bank Publications.

Smith, K. E. & Eltanani, M. K., 2015. What kinds of policies to reduce health inequalities in the UK do researchers support?. *Journal of Public Health,* 37(1), pp. 6-17.

Turkentine, R., 2010. *The London Health Inequality Strategy.* London: Evolution Satin.

Urquieta-Salomón, J. E. & Villarreal, H. J., 2015. Evolution of health coverage in Mexico: evidence of progress and challenges in the Mexican health system. *Health Policy Plan,* 31(1), pp. 28-36.

WHO, W. H. O., 2016. *Closing the Health Inequalities Gap: An International Perspective.* Copenhagen: WHO Regional Office for Europee.

Williamson A, 2020. Bridging the gap: an economic case study of the impact and cost effectiveness of comprehensive healthcare intermediaries in rural Mexico.. *Health Res Policy System,* pp. 68-75.

YOUR KNOWLEDGE HAS VALUE

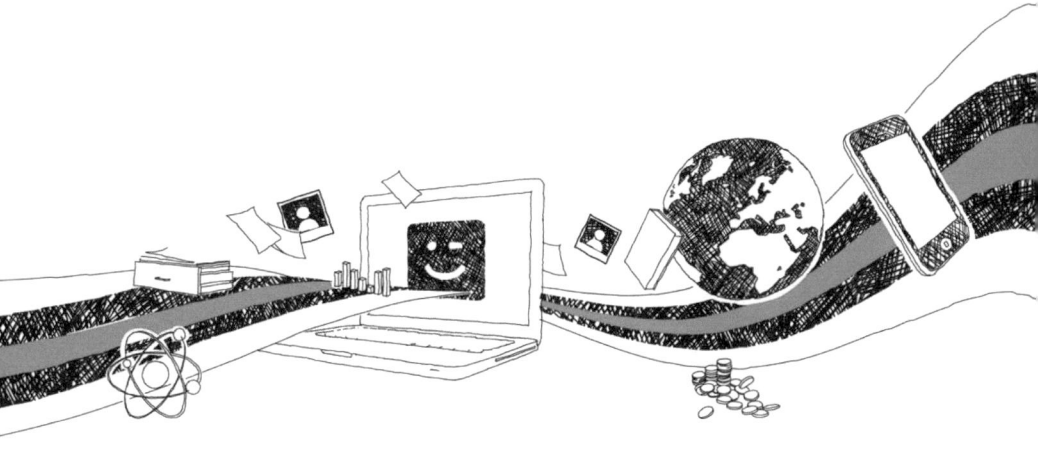

- We will publish your bachelor's and
  master's thesis, essays and papers

- Your own eBook and book -
  sold worldwide in all relevant shops

- Earn money with each sale

Upload your text at www.GRIN.com
and publish for free

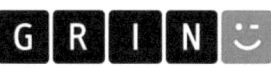